THE BAHÁ'Í FAITH AND FOOD

The Diet of the Future

GRACE J. KEENE, JD

Cover © Grace J. Keene via Canva.com
For permissions contact:
Grace J. Keene
Email: keenegracejauthor@gmail.com
Print ISBN: 9781658310413
Neither the publisher nor the author is engaged in rendering professional advice or services to the individual reader. The ideas, procedures, and suggestions contained in this book are not the substitute for consulting with your physician. All matters regarding your health require medical supervision. Neither the author nor the publisher shall be liable or responsible for any loss or damage allegedly arising from any information or suggestion in this book.

The author has made every effort to ensure the accuracy of the information within this book was correct at time of publication. The author does not assume and hereby disclaims any liability to any party for any loss, damage, or disruption caused by content, errors, or omissions, whether such content, errors, or omissions, result from accident, negligence, or any other cause.

Disclosure of Material Connection: The author has not received compensation from any party in connection with website links in this book.

❈ Created with Vellum

ABOUT THE AUTHOR

Grace J. Keene is an emerging author. She has baccalaureate degrees in Religion and Philosophy from Rutgers University and a JD from Widener University School of Law.

Grace has also written:

The Bahá'í Faith and Aliens: The Evidence Revealed

PROLOGUE

Humanity is creating consciousness that diet is directly related to health. Upon the rise in chronic disease, many people have turned to diet as a cure and palliative. These dietary remedies span a vast range and there is much uncertainty as to which option to choose.

Every major religion has given specific dietary guidelines tailored to humanity's physical and spiritual needs for each era. The Bahá'í Faith is one religion.

This new and rapidly growing world religion states that this dietary guidance throughout history comes from one God. The Bahá'í Faith states that all religions' sacred Founders are the divine Physicians for humanity. They cure society's and individuals' ills for each historical period. Thus, through diet, a person may achieve lasting physical and spiritual health.

There also have been accounts of near miraculous effects from certain diets. Some have cured terrible diseases, had increased longevity, and even spiritual awakening as a result of food, drink, and fasting.

Now, for the first time ever, the Bahá'í Faith reveals the diet of the future.

✣ I ✣

DIET AND RELIGION

Since time immemorial, people have turned to religion for guidance regarding what they should eat.

Christianity and Judaism are examples that have prescribed dietary guidelines for their adherents. For example, the Biblical book of Ezekiel prescribes wheat, barley, beans, and lentils.[1] The context suggests that this diet was a punishment but these grains are also healthy and may have been prescribed as a healing.

Leviticus says to avoid animal fat and blood and sets forth clean and unclean foods.[2] Jews are permitted to eat kosher food. Kosher means foods that have been prepared by Jewish law.

Further East, many Hindus are vegetarian or lacto-vegetarian (vegetarians who consume milk).[3] Those who are not avoid beef.

Buddhists are mostly vegetarian. Some others eat fish and naturally raised animal products.

Islam is another religion that contains dietary requirements for its adherents. The Qur'án prohibits carrion, blood, pork, and the meat of animals sacrificed "in the name of other than God."[4] The Qur'án prescribes instead fruits such as grapes, dates, olives, pomegranates, and "crops varying in taste."[5]

The Bahá'í Faith is a world religion that has prescribed dietary guidelines also. Bahá'u'lláh, the Founder of the Bahá'í Faith, revealed that religions are one and proceed from one God. Religions are a continuum where each religion has brought guidance to humanity from God.

One of those guidances has been diet. Diet always has historically featured in religion. This is no coincidence, because the Bahá'í Faith teaches that all religions come from the same God.

The reason some of the teachings differ is because they address different historical periods. Thus, dietary guidelines may differ due to the historical variances in what foods are available, the human body, what diseases exist at that point in history, the amount of exercise individuals would get, and other lifestyle concerns. This is a practical aspect that the Bahá'í concept of progressive revelation explains: that God's "medicine" or teachings for humanity must vary somewhat because the historical periods are so different. These small variances in religious beliefs are called the non-essential teachings.

However, *most of the teachings of these great religions are essentially the same*. They ask us to show forth love, compassion, trustworthiness, honesty, generosity, diligence, and other virtues that are familiar to everyone. Thus, these teachings are termed the essential teachings because they form the essence of the one ongoing religion of God.

THIS BOOK WILL EXPLORE WHAT THE BAHÁ! í FAITH PRESCRIBES AS its dietary guidelines, including whether or not to eat meat, fasting, modern dietary choices, and even the Faith's views on medical marijuana.

The Bahá'í Faith contains ten main teachings. These are:

"1. INDEPENDENT INVESTIGATION OF REALITY

Discover for yourselves the reality of things, and strive to assimilate the methods by which noble-mindedness and glory are attained among the nations and people of the world.

No man should follow blindly his ancestors and forefathers. Nay, each must see with his own eyes, hear with his own ears and investigate independently in order that he may find the truth. The religion of forefathers and ancestors is based upon blind imitation. Man should investigate reality.

2. ABANDONMENT OF ALL PREJUDICE

O people, make firm the girdle of endeavor, that perchance religious prejudice may be annulled. For love of God and his servants engage in this great and mighty matter. Religious hatred and rancor is a world-consuming fire, and the quenching thereof most arduous, unless the hand of divine might give men deliverance from this unfruitful calamity.

Beware of prejudice; light is good in whatsoever lamp it is burning. A rose is beautiful in whatever garden it may bloom. A star has the same radiance if it shines from the east or the west.

All the prophets of God have come to unite the children of men and not to disperse them; to put in action the law of love and not enmity.

We must banish prejudice. Religious, patriotic, racial prejudices must disappear, for they are the destroyers of human society.

We must become the cause of the unity of the human race.

3. THE ONENESS OF THE WORLD OF HUMANITY

White doves and gray doves associate with each other in perfect friendship. Man draws imaginary lines on the planet and says, 'This is a Frenchman, a Mussulman, an Italian!' Upon these differences wars are waged. Men are fighting for the possession of the earth. They fight for that which becomes their graves, their cemeteries, their tombs.

In reality all are members of one human family — children of one Heavenly Father. Humanity may be likened unto the vari-colored flowers of one garden. There is unity in diversity. Each sets off and enhances the other's beauty.

4. THE FOUNDATION OF ALL RELIGIONS IS ONE

The foundation underlying all the divine precepts is one reality. It must needs be reality and reality is one. Therefore the foundation of the divine religions is one. But we can see that certain forms and ceremonies have crept in. They are heretical, they are accidental, because they differ, hence they cause differences among religions. If we set aside all superstitions and seek the reality of the foundation we shall all agree, because religion is one and not multiple.

5. RELIGION MUST BE IN ACCORD WITH SCIENCE AND REASON

Religion must agree with science, so that science shall sustain religion and religion explain science. The two must be brought together, indissolubly, in reality. Down to the present day it has been customary for man to accept blindly what was called religion, even though it were not in accord with human reason. According to the Bahá'í Faith we do not need to do this anymore.

6. A UNIVERSAL LANGUAGE

A universal language shall be adopted and taught in the schools and academies of the world. A committee appointed by national bodies shall select a suitable language to be used as a means of international communication.

Every one will need but two languages, his national tongue and the universal language. All will acquire the universal language.

7. UNIVERSAL EDUCATION

Partaking of knowledge and education is one of the requisites of religion. The education of each child is obligatory. If there are no parents, the community must look after the child. It is suggested that the childless educate a child.

It is incumbent on every one to engage in some occupation, such as arts, trades, and the like. We have made this — your occupation — identical with the worship of God, the true one. Reflect, O people, upon the mercy of God, and upon his favors, then thank him in mornings and evenings.

8. EQUALITY BETWEEN MEN AND WOMEN

This is peculiar to the teachings of Bahá'u'lláh. Former religious systems placed men above women. In this new Dispensation, daughters and sons must follow the same form of study and acquire a uniform education. One course of education promotes unity among men and women.

9. AN INTERNATIONAL TRIBUNAL

The true civilization will raise its banner when some noble kings of high ambitions, the bright suns of the world of humanitarian enthusiasm, shall, for the good and happiness of all the human race, step forth with firm resolution and keen mind and hold a conference on the question of universal peace; when keeping fast hold of the means of enforcing their views they shall establish a union of the states of the world, and conclude a definite treaty and strict alliance between them upon conditions not to be evaded. When the whole human race has been consulted through their representatives and invited to corroborate this treaty which verily will be accounted sacred by all the peoples of the earth, it will be the duty of the united powers of the world to see that this great treaty shall endure.

A reflection of this parliament of man will be established in each community and called the 'house of justice.' Its members will be chosen for their attribute of justice, and all matters pertaining to the community interests will be brought here for consultation.

This Tribunal has already been elected and it represents the people of the world. It is called the Universal House of Justice. The House of Justice is now part of the Bahá'í Administrative Order. It manages the affairs of the Faith without ordaining clergy. A worldwide election process choses its members who serve for five years.[6]

10. UNIVERSAL PEACE

All men and nations shall make peace. There shall be universal peace amongst governments, universal peace amongst religions, universal peace amongst races, universal peace amongst the denizens of all regions. Today in the world of humanity the most important matter is the question of universal peace."[7]

Yes, this is a religion. Yet, the teachings are simple, practical, and elegant. Bahá'í believe that these teachings are divinely ordained. If implemented, they could change the world drastically for the better and pave the way for a new era in human history. At the present time, this new era has already begun with the implementation of the Bahá'í Teachings.[8]

---

1. Society of Biblical Literature, Wayne A. Meeks, ed., *The HarperCollins Study Bible: New Revised Standard Version With the Apocryphal/Deuterocanonical Books* (San Fransisco: HarperCollins, 1993), 1228-1229.

2. Ibid, 156, 167-169.

3. Susan Dudek, *Nutrition Essentials for Nursing Practice*, (Philadelphia: Wolters Kluwer Health, 2013), 251.

4. *The Qur'án: with Annotated Interpretation in Modern English*, trans. Ali Ünal, (Marquis, Canada: Tughra, 2015), 81.

5. Ibid, 304.

6. For more on this subject, see https://www.bahai.org/beliefs/essential-relationships/.administrative-order/.

7. 'Abdu'l-Bahá, *Abdul Baha On Divine Philosophy* (Boston: The Tudor Press, 1918), 25-27.

8. For more on these teachings, visit the official website: https://www.bahai.org.

✣ 2 ✣

THE NEW MEDICINE: FOOD

Bahá'u'lláh's Son and Official Interpreter, 'Abdu'l-Bahá, has explained that many human sicknesses result from a combination of improper diet and behavior.

"But man hath perversely continued to serve his lustful appetites, and he would not content himself with simple foods. Rather, he prepared for himself food that was compounded of many ingredients, of substances differing one from the other. With this, and with the perpetrating of vile and ignoble acts, his attention was engrossed, and he abandoned the temperance and moderation of a natural way of life. The result was the engendering of diseases both violent and diverse."[1]

Thus, temperance and moderation are familiar teachings from other religions. Also, the idea that compound foods with many ingredients can be harmful is a familiar one now, with the organic and natural food movement, and this text by 'Abdu'l-Bahá is from over 100 years ago. Thus, this point may be carried over in into dietary choices. However, the idea that lack of morality can cause disease is one that has not been widely acknowledged in modern times.

'Abdu'l-Bahá then goes on to compare humans with animals in this instance, saying that animals are relatively free of disease. He appears to suggest that this is because animals eat simple foods and commit "no sins." According to 'Abdu'l-Bahá, animals do not have free will, so they do not have morality. Instead they have instinct, where they obey natural law, their ecosystems's law. These ecosystems are balanced and can survive for thousands of years if uninterrupted. Thus, animals may be healthier because they are in harmony with nature. They also eat "simple foods." This is their "diet." Could 'Abdu'l-Bahá be suggesting that humans should eat a simple diet as well?

"For the animal, as to its body, is made up of the same constituent elements as man. Since, however, the animal contenteth itself with simple foods and striveth not to indulge its importunate urges to any great degree, and **committeth no sins**, its ailments relative to man's are few. We see clearly, therefore, how powerful are sin and contumacy as pathogenic factors. And once engendered these diseases become compounded, multiply, and are transmitted to others. Such are the spiritual, inner causes of sickness.

"The outer, physical causal factor in disease, however, **is a disturbance in the balance**, the proportionate equilibrium of all those elements of which the human body is composed. To illustrate: the body of man is a compound of many constituent substances, each component being present in a prescribed amount, contributing to the essential equilibrium of the whole. So long as these constituents remain in their due proportion, **according to the natural balance of the whole** — that is, no component suffereth a change in its natural proportionate degree and balance, no component being either augmented or decreased — there will be no physical cause for the incursion of disease.

"For example, the starch component must be present to a given amount, and the sugar to a given amount. So long as each remaineth in its natural proportion to the whole, there will be no cause for the onset of disease. When, however, these constituents vary as to their natural and due amounts — that is, when they are augmented or diminished — it is certain that this will provide for the inroads of disease."[2]

In modern terms, 'Abdu'l-Bahá appears to be referencing the body's homeostasis, or the proper internal balance. 'Abdu'l-Bahá also may be referring to holism, the idea that the human body must be treated as a whole and not as separate parts. This idea is familiar in ancient religions and medical systems.

The Báb is the Forerunner of the Bahá'í Revelation, akin to John the Baptist in the Christian context. The Báb has also suggested that foods can heal:

"This question requireth the most careful investigation. The Báb hath said that the people of Bahá must **develop the science of medicine to such a high degree that they will heal illnesses by means of foods. The basic reason for this is that if, in some component substance of the human body, an imbalance should occur, altering its correct, relative proportion to the whole, this fact will inevitably result in the onset of disease.** If, for example, the starch component should be unduly augmented, or the sugar component decreased, an illness will take control. It is the function of a skilled physician to determine which constituent of his patient's body hath suffered diminution, which hath been augmented. Once he hath discovered this, he must prescribe a food containing the diminished element in considerable amounts, **to re-establish the body's essential equilibrium.** The patient, once his constitution is again in balance, will be rid of his disease."[3]

'Abdu'l-Bahá then implies that animals already sense the relationship between food and health, and even use herbal medicine to cure themselves of disease:

"The proof of this is that while other animals have never studied medical science, nor carried on researches into diseases or medicines, treatments or cures — even so, when one of them falleth a prey to sickness, nature leadeth it, in fields or desert places, to the very plant which, once eaten, will rid the animal of its disease. The explanation is that if, as an example, the sugar component in the animal's body hath decreased, according to a natural law the animal hankereth after a herb that is rich in sugar. **Then, by a natural urge, which is the appetite, among a thousand different varieties of plants across the field, the animal will discover and consume that herb** which containeth a sugar component in large amounts. Thus the essential balance of the substances composing its body is re-established, and **the animal is rid of its disease**."[4]

The holistic approach says that the body must be treated as a whole. Also, the body's substances (or "humors" as we shall see in the last chapter, the energetic component of this) must be proportionate to maintain homeostasis. Food intake can control this balance. So, according to the Bahá'í Faith the medical science will eventually advance until people can cure disease through diet.

"This question requireth the most careful investigation. When highly-skilled physicians shall fully examine this matter, thoroughly and perseveringly, **it will be clearly seen that the incursion of disease is due to a disturbance in the relative amounts of the body's component substances, and that treatment consisteth in adjusting these relative amounts, and that this can be apprehended and made possible by means of foods**.

"**It is certain that in this wonderful new age the development of medical science will lead to the doctors' healing their patients with foods.** For the sense of sight, the sense of hearing, of taste, of smell, of touch — all these are discriminative faculties, their purpose being to separate the beneficial from whatever causeth harm. Now, is it possible that man's sense of smell, the sense that differentiates odours, should find some odour repugnant, and that odour be beneficial to the human body? Absurd! Impossible! In the same way, could the human body, through the faculty of sight — the differentiator among things visible — benefit from gazing upon a revolting mass of excrement? Never! Again, if the sense of taste, likewise a faculty that selecteth and rejecteth, be offended by something, that thing is certainly not beneficial; and if, at the outset, it may yield some advantage, in the long run its harmfulness will be established.

"And likewise, when the constitution is in a state of equilibrium, there is no doubt that whatever is relished will be beneficial to health. Observe how an animal will graze in a field where there are a hundred thousand kinds of herbs and grasses, and how, with its sense of smell, it snuffeth up the odours of the plants, and tasteth them with its sense of taste; then it consumeth whatever herb is pleasurable to these senses, and benefitteth therefrom. Were it not for this power of selectivity, the animals would all be dead in a single day; for there are a great many poisonous plants, and animals know nothing of the pharmacopoeia. And yet, observe what a reliable set of scales they have, by means of which to differentiate the good from the injurious. Whatever constituent of their body hath decreased, they can rehabilitate by seeking out and consuming some plant that hath an abundant store of that diminished element; and thus the equilibrium of their bodily components is re-established, and they are rid of their disease.

"At whatever time highly-skilled physicians shall have developed the healing of illnesses by means of foods, and shall make provision for simple foods, and shall prohibit humankind from living as slaves to their lustful appetites, it is certain that the incidence of chronic and diversified illnesses will abate, and the general health of all mankind will be much improved. This is destined to come about. In the same way, in the character, the conduct and the manners of men, universal modifications will be made."[5]

Could 'Abdu'l-Bahá be referring to herbal medicine? He also appears to say that diet itself is the way to cure and control disease and that spirituality is a key component to physical and mental health.

MEDICAL CARE, DRUGS AND ALCOHOL

IN THE BAHÁ! Í FAITH'S MOST HOLY BOOK, THE KITÁB-I-AQDAS, Bahá'u'lláh, prescribes exactly what Bahá'ís believe God ordained for humanity at this time.

First, Bahá'u'lláh states that, when ill, competent medical care is important.

"Resort ye, in times of sickness, to competent physicians; We have not set aside the use of material means, rather have We confirmed it through this Pen, which God has made to be the Dawning-place of His shining and glorious Cause."[6]

Thus, the Bahá'í Faith teaches the reconciliation of science and religion. Under this tenet, Bahá'ís are encouraged to use reason and logic in their spiritual pursuits and embrace scientific fact.

This truth can be reflected in the Bahá'í Faith's prohibition of recreational alcohol and drugs. These substances impair reason, without which humanity may not progress spiritually:

"It is inadmissible that man, who hath been endowed with reason, should consume that which stealeth it away. Nay, rather it behoveth him to comport himself in a manner worthy of the human station, and not in accordance with the misdeeds of every heedless and wavering soul."[7]

The explanation in the notes in the Kitáb-i-Aqdas states that this prohibition goes for anything that intoxicates and deranges the mind. However, **a qualified physician may use alcohol and other intoxicants to heal the patient**:

"There are many references in the Bahá'í Writings which prohibit the use of wine and other intoxicating drinks and which describe the deleterious effect of such intoxicants on the individual. In one of His Tablets, Bahá'u'lláh states:

'Beware lest ye exchange the Wine of God for your own wine, for it will stupefy your minds, and turn your faces away from the Countenance of God, the All-Glorious, the Peerless, the Inaccessible. Approach it not, for it hath been forbidden unto you by the behest of God, the Exalted, the Almighty.

"'Abdu'l-Bahá explains that the Aqdas [the Most Holy Book] prohibits 'both light and strong drinks', and He states that the reason for prohibiting the use of alcoholic drinks is because 'alcohol leadeth the mind astray and causeth the weakening of the body.'

"Shoghi Effendi, in letters written on his behalf, states that this prohibition includes not only the consumption of wine but of 'everything that derangeth the mind,' and he clarifies that the use of alcohol is permitted only when it constitutes part of a medical treatment which is implemented 'under the advice of a competent and conscientious physician, who may have to prescribe it for the cure of some special ailment."[8]

This prohibition also applies to opium, LSD and other drugs.

"Gambling and the use of opium have been forbidden unto you. Eschew them both, O people, and be not of those who transgress. Beware of using any substance that induceth sluggishness and torpor in the human temple and inflicteth harm upon the body. We, verily, desire for you naught save what shall profit you, and to this bear witness all created things, had ye but ears to hear."[9]

This opium prohibition is so important that the Kitáb-i-Aqdas ends with a final warning:

"It hath been forbidden you to smoke opium. We, truly, have prohibited this practice through a most binding interdiction in the Book. Should anyone partake thereof, assuredly he is not of Me."[10]

In this connection, Shoghi Effendi stated that one of the requirements for 'a chaste and holy life' is 'total abstinence ... from opium, and from **similar habit-forming drugs**.'

"Heroin, hashish and other **derivatives of cannabis such as marijuana,** as well as hallucinogenic agents such as **LSD**, **peyote** and similar substances, are regarded as falling under this prohibition.

"'Abdu'l-Bahá has written:

"*As to opium, it is foul and accursed. God protect us from the punishment He inflicteth on the user. According to the explicit Text of the Most Holy Book, it is forbidden, and its use is utterly condemned. Reason showeth that smoking opium is a kind of insanity, and experience attesteth that the user is* **completely cut off from the human kingdom.** *May God protect all against the perpetration of an act so hideous as this, an act which layeth in ruins the very foundation of what it is to be human, and which causeth the user to be dispossessed for ever and ever. For opium fasteneth on the soul so that the user's conscience dieth, his mind is blotted away, his perceptions are eroded. It turneth the living into the dead. It quencheth the natural heat. No greater harm can be conceived than that which opium inflicteth. Fortunate are they who never even speak the name of it; then think how wretched is the user.*

"*O ye lovers of God! In this, the cycle of Almighty God, violence and force, constraint and oppression, are one and all condemned. It is, however, mandatory that the use of opium be prevented by any means whatsoever, that perchance the human race may be delivered from this most powerful of plagues. And otherwise, woe and misery to whoso falleth short of his duty to his Lord.*

"In one of His Tablets 'Abdu'l-Bahá has stated concerning opium: '*the user, the buyer and the seller are all deprived of the bounty and grace of God.*'

"In yet another Tablet, 'Abdu'l-Bahá has written:

"*Regarding* **hashish** *you have pointed out that some Persians have become* *habituated to its use. Gracious God! This is the worst of all intoxicants, and its prohibition is explicitly revealed. Its use causeth the disintegration of thought and the complete torpor of the soul. How could anyone seek the fruit of the infernal tree, and by partaking of it, be led to exemplify the qualities of a monster? How could one use this forbidden drug, and thus deprive himself of the blessings of the All-Merciful?"*[11]

The probable reason the Kitáb-i-Aqdas so strongly prohibited opium is because it was a pervasive problem at the time and highly addictive. Interestingly, more modern drugs like marijuana and LSD are also prohibited.

Alcohol has similar effects and this was the reason for its prohibition in the Kitáb-i-Aqdas:

"'Alcohol consumeth the mind and causeth man to commit acts of absurdity, but this opium, this foul fruit of the infernal tree, and this wicked hashish extinguish the mind, freeze the spirit, petrify the soul, waste the body and leave man frustrated and lost.'" [12]

Thus, the reasons for the prohibition are manifold and not merely because drugs and alcohol impair the senses. The harmful effects of drugs and alcohol are well known, but Bahá'u'lláh and 'Abdu'l-Bahá explain the spiritual reasons for this: that opium and other recreational drugs destroy *the human faculty of reason, the definition of what it is to be human.* In other words, they destroy the difference between the human and animal kingdoms. Humans are uniquely able to know and love God and are able to use reason. Animals cannot do this.[13]

Also, this extensive prohibition on recreational drugs and alcohol could be another indication that diet and consumption of foods and substances can affect human spiritual growth, an idea that previous religions may attest to in their dietary guidelines. Bahá'ís would agree that religious laws treat humanity's ills, thus diet is a part of this treatment.

CANNABIS, AND OTHER PLANTS AS MEDICINE

. . .

However, the Kitáb-i-Aqdas states in a note from paragraph 155 that **intoxicants are allowed as part of medical treatment:**

"It should be noted that the above prohibition against taking certain classes of drugs does not forbid their use when prescribed by qualified physicians as part of a medical treatment."[14] Kitáb-i-Aqdas specifies one herb in particular in this note: **cannabis**.

This note may have been foreseeing the medical use of cannabidiol, or CBD, a cannabis derivative that is not intoxicating. It has been alleged to be effective against a wide range of ailments. Studies have noted that CBD is an antispasmodic and anti-epileptic.[15] Others have alleged that CBD is an anti-inflammatory, analgesic, muscle relaxer, antidepressant, and immunity modulator.[16]

CBD is also alleged to be not addictive; it occurs naturally in the human body. Thus, it does not fall under the prohibition of intoxicants in the Kitáb-i-Aqdas. Humans and certain animals have receptors for CBD in their nervous systems.[17] The CBD helps regulate that system, thus promoting balance or homeostasis.[18] Thus, this herb (cannabis), may be a natural alternative for disease treatment that the Kitáb-i-Aqdas allows.

In addition, herbalists use potential intoxicants in non-intoxicating quantities. For example, many herbalists create preparations using alcohol. These are called tinctures. The herbalist soaks the raw herb in alcohol for a number of weeks while the alcohol extracts the chemical compounds from the plant. The raw plant is then strained out from the alcohol, leaving the liquefied chemical compounds from the plant material and the alcohol. This is the finished tincture, which the patient may take in doses as small as one drop.[19] **Hemp** is a form of cannabis that contains less than 0.03% of THC.[20] Herbalists may prepare CBD in the above method as tinctures using a variety of extractors such as coconut oil. Many of these preparations are organic. Organic means they are made without genetically engineered organisms or GMOs and other impurities like pesticides, artificial fertilizers, etc. The simpler preparations also are full-spectrum, meaning that all of the compounds in the plant are included in the preparation. This is important because the active compound, the "isolate" if prepared in a laboratory, is more effective when taken *with* the other compounds in the plant.

Thus, there is a wealth of knowledge that that Bahá'í Faith reveals. **The Bahá'í Faith allows for diet as a treatment for illness. The Faith also asserts that spiritual conduct affects physical health and vice-versa.**

Also, *there are virtual prophecies of what the medical world will be in the future: where disease will be cured by diet, liquids, and herbs.* In the next chapter we shall see in more detail what the human body demands by way of nutrition.

---

1. 'Abdu'l-Bahá, *Writings and Utterances of 'Abdu'l-Bahá*, ed. (Wilmette: Bahá'í Publishing Trust, 2000), 378.
2. Ibid.
3. Ibid, 379.
4. Ibid.
5. Ibid 379-380.
6. Bahá'u'lláh, *The Kitáb-i-Aqdas: The Most Holy Book*, (Haifa: Bahá'í World Centre, 1992), 60.
7. Ibid, 62.
8. Ibid, 226-227, n. 144.
9. Ibid, 75.
10. Ibid, 88.
11. Ibid, 238-239, n. 170.
12. Ibid.
13. 'Abdu'l-Bahá, *Some Answered Questions*, trans. Newly Revised by a Committee at the Bahá'í World Centre, (Wilmette: Bahá'í Publishing Trust, 2014), 273-280.
14. Bahá'u'lláh, *The Kitáb-i-Aqdas*, 239, n. 170.
15. Craig Tomashoff, "To CBD or Not to CBD?," *Centennial Spotlight*, 2019.
16. Ibid.
17. Ibid.
18. Ibid.
19. Matthew Wood, *The Book of Herbal Wisdom: Using Plants as Medicines*, (Berkeley: North Atlantic Books, 1997), 59-60.
20. Tomashoff, "To CBD or Not to CBD?"

⚛ 3 ⚛

TO EAT OR NOT TO EAT MEAT?

‘Abdu'l-Bahá, the Official Interpreter of Bahá'u'lláh, explains that humans are suited to vegan foods. 'Abdu'l-Bahá says that the shape of our teeth is one indicator of this. Another indicator is the health of the people who consume this diet:

"But now coming to man, we see he hath neither hooked teeth nor sharp nails or claws, nor teeth like iron sickles. From this it becometh evident and manifest that the food of man is cereals and fruit. Some of the teeth of man are like millstones to grind the grain, and some are sharp to cut the fruit. Therefore he is not in need of meat, nor is he obliged to eat it. Even without eating meat he would live with the utmost vigour and energy. For example, the community of the Brahmins in India do not eat meat; notwithstanding this they are not inferior to other nations in strength, power, vigour, outward senses or intellectual virtues. Truly, the killing of animals and the eating of their meat is somewhat contrary to pity and compassion, and if one can content oneself with cereals, fruit, oil and nuts, such as pistachios, almonds and so on, it would undoubtedly be better and more pleasing."[1]

Thus, 'Abdu'l-Bahá suggests that humans are frugivores. 'Abdu'l-Bahá also adds:

"Thou hast written regarding the four canine teeth in man, saying that these teeth, two in the upper jaw and two in the lower, are for the purpose of eating meat. Know thou that these four teeth are not created for meat-eating, although one can eat meat with them. All the teeth of man are made for eating fruit, cereals and vegetables. These four teeth, however, are designed for breaking hard shells, such as those of almonds."[2]

Thus, 'Abdu'l-Bahá says that the four canine teeth are for eating nuts. Shoghi Effendi echoes the idea that people should eat plant-based diets while also encouraging debate on dietary choices:

"In regard to the question as to whether people ought to kill animals for food or not, there is no explicit statement in the Bahá'í Sacred Scriptures (as far as I know) in favour or against it. It is certain, however, that if man can live on a purely vegetarian diet and thus avoid killing animals, it would be much preferable. This is, however, a very controversial question and the Bahá'ís are free to express their views on it."[3]

HOWEVER, EATING MEAT IS ALLOWED IN THE BAHÁ'Í FAITH. THIS is partly because it may be necessary in some circumstances:

"But eating meat is not forbidden or unlawful, nay the point is this, that it is possible for man to live without eating meat and still be strong. Meat is nourishing and containeth the elements of herbs, seeds and fruits; therefore sometimes it is essential for the sick and for the rehabilitation of health. There is no objection in the Law of God to the eating of meat if it is required. So if thy constitution is rather weak and thou findest meat useful, thou mayest eat it."[4]

Bahá'u'lláh, the Founder of the Faith encourages vegetarianism, while at the same time giving freedom to eat meat especially where this is necessary for survival. In addition, while there are no express prohibitions on meat consumption, Bahá'ís are required to show kindness to animals. Bahá'u'lláh says:

"As in so many other areas, the Teachings of Bahá'u'lláh in this regard follow the golden mean: kindness toward animals is definitely upheld, vegetarianism is encouraged, hunting is regulated, but certain latitude is left to individual conscience and in practical regard to the diversity of circumstances under which human beings live. For example, the indigenous peoples of the Arctic would be hard-pressed to subsist without recourse to animal products."[5]

This is similar to the dietary laws from previous religions, that was covered in the Prologue, suggest that the religions of the past have leaned toward vegetarian foods over animal food. They did not prohibit meat, but carved out exceptions for its consumption and encouraged adherents to eat fruits and grains.

Regarding hunting, Bahá'u'lláh states in the Kitáb-i-Aqdas that hunting for food is allowed for Bahá'ís if done with moderation and respect:

"If ye should hunt with beasts or birds of prey, invoke ye the Name of God when ye send them to pursue their quarry; for then whatever they catch shall be lawful unto you, even should ye find it to have died. [. . .] Take heed, however, that ye hunt not to excess. Tread ye the path of justice and equity in all things."[6]

The Universal House of Justice has also explained that meat is not prohibited and may be necessary in places where fruits and vegetables are unobtainable.

Thus, Bahá'ís are permitted to try different food choices. 'Abdu'l-Bahá has explained that, in the future, humans will rely more and more on vegan foods.

"'What will be the food of the future?' Fruit and grains. The time will come when meat will no longer be eaten. Medical science is only in its infancy, yet it has shown that our natural diet is that which grows out of the ground. The people will gradually develop up to the condition of this natural food."[7]

Finally, 'Abdu'l-Bahá links this diet to humanity's progress. Could He be suggesting that this transition to a vegan diet is part of human evolution?

---

1. Compiled by Ernie Jones, *Bahá'í Teachings on Health Healing and Nutrition: A compilation of compilations from online sources arranged by subject*, (2017), 8.
2. Ibid.
3. Ibid, 9.

4. Compiled by the Research Department of The Universal House of Justice, *Health and Healing*, (New Delhi: Bahá'í Publishing Trust, 2004), 8-9.

5. Jones, 9.

6. Bahá'u'lláh, *The Kitáb-i-Aqdas*, 40.

7. 'Abdu'l-Bahá, cited in Julia M. Grundy, *Ten Days in the Light of 'Akka*, rev. ed. (Wilmette: Bahá'í Publishing Trust, 1979) 8-9.

❧ 4 ❧

WHICH DIET IS RIGHT FOR YOU?

There are many views on which diet is good for the human being. This determination may vary based numerous factors like the following:

1. **Region**. A key factor in dietary choice is region. As the Bahá'í Faith suggests, allowances should be made for climate and food availability. As the Universal House of Justice has explained, living in extremely cold climates would be nearly impossible without meat consumption, for example. Other areas may have other environmental factors that would alter the inhabitants' dietary needs.

2. **Historical Period**. Historical period is another factor in the determination. In the past, humans have had access to only the food choices available in their respective regions. In the future, when foods become more available, people may transition to diets that better suit the human genome independent of the geographical.

3. **Health**. Finally, health is the final determination. What foods are healthier? This is the most debatable subject.

Thus, the proposed diets range from the ketogenic diet where much fat is consumed, to strictly vegan, which requires no animal products. Vegan diets are sub-categorized into many niches such as lacto-vegan, ovo-vegan, and raw vegan. This chapter will discuss the ketogenic, paleolithic, anti-inflammatory, vegetarian, vegan, raw vegan diets, with the above factors in mind. Keep in mind that Bahá'ís are allowed to make their own dietary choices. This is in tandem with previous religions such as Islam and Christianity, where there were few prohibitions but many suggestions. Eastern religions have an entire dietary science, which is beyond this book's scope.

'Abdu'l-Bahá in *Some Answered Questions* suggests that a vegan diet is healthier, if possible, for the person to adhere to:

"The science of medicine is still in its infancy and has not yet reached maturity. But when it reaches that stage, treatments will be administered with things that are not repulsive to the senses of taste and smell, that is, through food, fruits, and plants that have an agreeable taste and pleasant smell."[1]

We saw the progression in dietary religious laws in this book's Prologue. Those ancient diets carried suggestions that vegan foods are better for the human constitution. According to the Bahá'í Faith, humanity is at a transitional stage.

PALEOLITHIC DIET: ANCIENT HUMANITY

SCIENTISTS HAVE DETERMINED WHAT EARLY HUMANS ATE FROM examining their remains and from determining what flora and fauna humans could consume at this early part of human history. Physiologist Loren Cordain popularized the diet as what early hunter-gatherers would eat.

The diet generally consists of fruits and vegetables, nuts, tubers, and meat. Foods that paleo dieters avoid are generally, dairy products such as cheese and yogurt, grains, sugar, legumes, processed oils, salt, alcohol, and coffee.

Detractors claim that humans have changed since the time of early humanity, making our nutritional needs different. This, however, is not true. In addition, the diet was designed to mimic the adaptability that early hunter-gatherers would have needed to survive day-to-day in uncertain times.

This diet partially agrees with Bahá'í scripture in that the foods are required to be as pure and as unprocessed as possible. This is because the paleolithic diet is modeled after what humans would have allegedly been eating in the paleolithic era before agriculture. Thus, humans were eating unprocessed food.

As we saw in chapter 1, Bahá'í scripture suggests that purer, simpler foods are healthier. Thus, under this diet, artificial chemicals, genetically modified organisms (GMOs), and other contaminants would potentially be discouraged. Foods that do not allow for these alleged contaminants are labelled "organic."

Additionally, there is the regional concern. Author Aqiyl Aniys has written in his book, *Alkaline Herbal Medicine,* that the reason humans trace their genetic roots to Africa is that the African continent contained food choices that were uniquely suited to the human genome.[2] This is not surprising, since mitochondrial DNA in humans suggests that humans originated from Africa. Apparently, the African soil contained a richness that could support tremendous biodiversity, especially in plants. As humanity spread elsewhere, it brought the healthy genome from its birthplace: Africa.

Many African plants have medicinal qualities that enable the few untouched tribes to treat their own diseases internally without hospitals or trained doctors. This feat would be almost inconceivable in the "modern" world.

KETOGENIC DIET: "WEIGHT LOSS THROUGH FAT Consumption"

THE KETOGENIC DIET ORIGINATED AS A TREATMENT FOR EPILEPSY IN children, but people have now popularized it as a method for weight loss. The idea is that if a person increases his or her fat intake and reduce carbohydrate intake, it would trick the body into rapid, dramatic weight loss. The problem with this, however, is: what happens to the body's internal balance afterwards?

The Bahá'í Writings suggest that the body requires an internal balance of substances to maintain homeostasis. Under this advice then, the ketogenic diet may prove problematic.

Region may also be an issue here because colder temperatures mean more calories burned and fat contains more calories than other types of food. Thus, in a colder climate, the ketogenic diet might have less of an impact. However, typically people who live in arctic climates already consume the proper diet for the region.

Historical period is also relevant. The Bible banned eating animal fat. The Qur'án banned eating pork, one of the meats with the highest fat content. Eastern religions tend to favor vegetarianism. Therefore, the ketogenic diet would be one that these religions would disfavor.

ANTI-INFLAMMATORY DIET: DO NOT "INFLAME" THE BODY.

AS THE TITLE SUGGESTS, THE ANTI-INFLAMMATORY DIET ATTEMPTS to reduce inflammation in the body. This inflammation results from arachidonic acid from different foods.[3] Some claim that inflammation in the body causes many human disorders.

The diet includes: organic fruits, vegetables, legumes, nuts, seeds and whole grains, eggs, herbal teas, and lighter meats like chicken and fish.[4] It omits: red meat, fried foods, wheat, sugar and artificial sweeteners, refined foods, white rice, dairy products, peanuts, soft drinks, coffee, chocolate, and alcohol, all of which supporters of this diet link with inflammation.[5]

Some people are already using diet to control disease. For example, in her book *Healing Depression & Bipolar Disorder Without Drugs: Inspiring Stories of Restoring Mental Health Through Natural Therapies,* Gracelyn Guyol presents her story of having alleviated her bipolar symptoms through diet and other natural therapies.[6]

People may lose weight on this diet due to omitting the fattening foods. As we saw in the first chapter, the cleaner and purer the food, organic, and unprocessed, allegedly the better it will be. The purpose is to maintain the body's equilibrium by removing poisons like pesticides and other chemicals from the diet.

Nonetheless, region may be a problem in trying to follow this diet, again because red meat is a very high percentage of what people in colder climates must consume to survive.

VEGETARIAN DIET: WHAT EASTERN RELIGIONS FAVOR

VEGETARIANISM INCLUDES EVERYTHING BUT MEAT, INCLUDING EGGS and dairy products. Much of the food is cooked, not raw, as in raw vegan diets which we will discuss below.

Supporters say this is healthy because plant foods contain many nutrients and because meat is acid-forming and too much acid is not good for the human body. The body's pH is something that affects the entire organism. It is easy to manipulate your pH through diet. You can measure your own pH with test strips that measure pH in both saliva and urine. The pH should be alkaline: 7.4 is optimal for saliva and blood.

Experts in the area have noted that body fluid alkalinity is vital for health. Natural chemical reactions in the body slow down in an acidic environment. The immune system is one that experts have asserted will not function properly if the blood pH is acidic. Thus, if this is true, by removing meat, you can take an almost gratuitous step in this direction because some acid-forming foods will have been eliminated.

One good way to control pH is to get a small guide with all of the acidifying and alkalizing foods listed and look up foods before consuming them.[7] Alkalizing foods will drive up the pH and the acidifying foods will lower it. You may test your saliva or urine every few days with the test strips until you get to the target pH.

A glass of fresh-squeezed lemon juice mixed with water and no sugar every morning is an effective alkalizer. Yes, lemons are acidic, but the body converts this acid into alkaline compounds in the body, so it becomes alkaline.

The drawback is that some vegetarians "compensate" by adding a lot of sugar, dairy, and wheat flour which are acid-forming. These foods may taste good but the key is moderation.

Religion has attested to this tenet of moderation as has the Bahá'í Faith. As shown in the previous chapters, Bahá'u'lláh and His Official Interpreter 'Abdu'l-Bahá have suggested moderation in all things including diet. Followers of other religions would agree with this tenet, too because it is an essential teaching of the religion of God.

Fermentation is another healthy choice that vegetarians and others take advantage of because it enhances flavor. The bacteria also aid the gut.

Fermentation is easy to get into as a hobby. Kefir, and yogurt are as easy as an overnight fermentation. Yogurt is particularly easy in that it is just a tablespoon of store-bought yogurt to a bowl of milk and an overnight wait in a warm room. In the morning, presto: more yogurt. Kombucha or fermented tea, takes about a week to make and is another healthy liquid.

VEGAN DIET: RAW OR NOT RAW?

VEGANISM HAS ENJOYED A METEORIC RISE IN THE NEW MILLENNIUM. The Bahá'í Faith encourages vegan food and is saying that veganism will be the diet of the future. Many religions have recommended, but not required, this diet.

Vegans eat only plant foods. There are vegans who also eliminate processed foods and wheat because they tend to be acid-forming.

Some vegans cook the foods and others eat only raw foods, thus are "raw vegans." Author and filmmaker Markus Rothkranz has written a guide on how to carry on a raw vegan diet: he asserts that raw plant foods are healthier because they include the natural enzymes in the plants that cooking kills.[8] Thus, raw foods are *"still alive."* These live enzymes are healthful in that they aid the chemical reactions in the body, giving it more energy.

Coupled with the alkalizing power of the plant foods, a raw vegan diet is allegedly healthy if you live in a temperate or warmer climate. Again, if you live in a colder one, you may have to supplement your diet with meat and high calorie foods. A possible drawback of this diet is protein deficiency, but many plant foods like beans, chickpeas, nuts and seeds are protein-rich.

Some people think that raw plant foods will be bland in taste. Think of it this way: try eating meat with no spices whatsoever. What does it taste like? (I think everybody has had that steak that someone forgot to marinate at the barbecue and made everybody mad because it tasted like, well, nothing.) That is because *most spices are plants*. Thus, the real flavor is in the plant side of the equation, not the meats. Good chefs know that the best spices are fresh and raw. They season the dishes with plant spices freshly cut after the dish is cooked to avoid wilting. Thus, anyone can make plant food taste however they want through putting spices on already flavor-rich plant dishes. Thus, there is a gamut of flavors to choose from.

Humans only eat a few species of animals, all of which taste dull without plants, while the plant varieties available as food are virtually endless. In addition, plant foods are cheaper to buy that meats, especially if you buy them fresh at the local farmers or asian markets, where the majority of the produce is organic, even though not labelled as such.

Cheese need not be eliminated, there are substitutes for vegan cheese at the store that taste similar. Nutritional yeast is another cheese substitute that is healthy and tastes similar to cheese.

In sum, this diet may be the diet that 'Abdu'l-Bahá says is the diet of the future. There are endless possibilities inherent in it, to keep the human body healthy, if you get sick to cure illness, and enhanced flavor.

While this chapter has discussed food, the next chapter will discuss abstinence from it: the wonderful world of *fasting*.

---

1. 'Abdu'l-Bahá, *Some Answered Questions*, trans. Newly Revised by a Committee at the Bahá'í World Centre, (Wilmette: Bahá'í Publishing Trust, 2014), 379.
2. Aqiyl Aniys, *Alkaline Herbal Medicine: Reverse Disease and Heal The Electric Body*, (North Charlston, SC: CreateSpace Independent Publishing Platform, 2016), 7.
3. Gracelyn Guyol, *Healing Depression & Bipolar Disorder Without Drugs: Inspiring Stories of Restoring Mental Health Through Natural Therapies*, (New York: Walker Publishing Company, 2006) 223.
4. Ibid, 223-224.

5. Ibid.

6. Ibid.

7. See for example: Susan E. Brown and Larry Trivieri Jr., *The Acid-Alkaline Food Guide - Second Edition: A Quick Reference to Foods and Their Effect on pH Levels,*

8. Markus Rothkranz, *Heal Yourself 101: Get Younger and Never Get Sick Again,* (Rothkranz Publishing, 2016).

BAHÁ'Í FASTING: WHEN, HOW,
WHY, AND WHO

"*Pen of the Most High! Say: O people of the world! We have enjoined upon you fasting during a brief period, and at its close have designated for you Naw-Rúz as a feast. Thus hath the Day-Star of Utterance shone forth above the horizon of the Book as decreed by Him Who is the Lord of the beginning and the end.*"[1]

WHEN AND HOW TO FAST?

IN HIS MOST HOLY BOOK, THE KITÁB-I-AQDAS, BAHÁ'U'LLÁH instructs to abstain from food, drink and smoking from sunrise to sunset for nineteen days.[2]

"In one of His Tablets, 'Abdu'l-Bahá, after stating that fasting consists of abstinence from food and drink, further indicates that smoking is a form of "drink". In Arabic the verb "drink" applies equally to smoking."[3]

Bahá'ís begin their fast at dawn and break their fast at sunset. Bahá'ís often awaken before dawn to have a light meal to lessen the impact of the twelve-hour fast. This period of fasting goes on for nineteen days, from March 2 to March 20. After the nineteen days, the Kitáb-i-Aqdas prescribes a feast called Naw-Rúz that inaugurates the new year. The celebration is a festive one with the fast broken at sunset along with music and dancing.

The purpose of the fast is spiritual development. Fasting enhances self-control. According to a prayer by 'Abdu'l-Bahá, for a person to develop spiritually, the body and soul must be purified of all impurities:

"O God! As my body has become purified and cleansed from physical impurities, in the same way purify and sanctify my spirit from the impurities of the world of nature, which are not worthy of the Threshold of Thy Unity!"[4]

This prayer suggests that bodily purification is important. Authors such as Markus Rothkranz, Arnold Ehret and others have claimed that fasting causes detoxification of the body. This is something that raw vegans may be familiar with because raw vegan food allegedly tends to produce similar effects. Thus, fasting may be one of the ways to purify the body and soul. This is in tandem with what Shoghi Effendi, Bahá'u'lláh's Grandson, explains: that the fast is "a period for meditation and prayer" for the person to regulate and heal his or her inner life and "recuperate" spiritually.

WHY FAST?

"FASTING AND OBLIGATORY PRAYER CONSTITUTE THE TWO PILLARS that sustain the revealed Law of God. Bahá'u'lláh in one of His Tablets affirms that He has revealed the laws of obligatory prayer and fasting so that through them the believers may draw nigh unto God.

Shoghi Effendi indicates in a note from the Kitáb-i-Aqdas that the fasting period, which involves complete abstention from food and drink from sunrise till sunset, is:

"' ...essentially a period of meditation and prayer, of spiritual recuperation, during which the believer must strive to make the necessary readjustments in his inner life, and to refresh and reinvigorate the spiritual forces latent in his soul. Its significance and purpose are, therefore, fundamentally spiritual in character. Fasting is symbolic, and a reminder of abstinence from selfish and carnal desires.'"[5]

Fasting is an ancient practice, one that even the Founders of many world religions engaged in. Jesus, Buddha, Muhammad, and Bahá'u'lláh all fasted at key junctures in Their ministries.

That the fast is symbolic is another point that suggests that dietary practices such as fasting may lead to spiritual development. This is because the physical act itself, abstaining from dood and drink for a period of time, is not itself symbolic. Rather, the spiritual component is presumably what is symbolic. Thus, the symbolism may be referring to something intangible like spiritual growth. This spiritual growth is often symbolically mentioned in sacred scripture because it is difficult to describe.

The Báb has stated that the fast is a time of abstaining from everything save love for the Promised One of all religions: Bahá'u'lláh.

Further, the Bahá'í calendar, where the fast appears, is steeped in ancient astronomy. The Kitáb-i-Aqdas explains:

"Naw-Rúz is the first day of the new year. It coincides with the spring equinox in the northern hemisphere, which usually occurs on 21 March. Bahá'u'lláh explains that this feast day is to be celebrated on whatever day the sun passes into the constellation of Aries, the vernal equinox, even should this occur one minute before sunset. Hence Naw-Rúz could fall on 20, 21, or 22 March, depending on the time of the equinox."[6]

Placing major events like the Bahá'í Naw-Rúz on the equinoxes is familiar in ancient calendars. Naw-Rúz also dates back to ancient times, before the Bahá'í Revelation.

The Bahá'í calendar contains five excess days, intercalary days, that should precede the fast. During those five days, called the Ayyám-i-Há celebration, the Most Holy Book urges Bahá'ís to pray, celebrate and practice charity as the "days of giving that precede the season of restraint."[7]

"Let the days in excess of the months be placed before the month of fasting. We have ordained that these, amid all nights and days, shall be the manifestations of the letter Há ("Essence of God") and, thus, they have not been bounded by the limits of the year and its months. It behoveth the people of Bahá, throughout these days, to provide good cheer for themselves, their kindred and, beyond them, the poor and needy, and with joy and exultation to hail and glorify their Lord, to sing His praise and magnify His Name; and when they end--these days of giving that precede the season of restraint--let them enter upon the Fast. Thus hath it been ordained by Him Who is the Lord of all mankind."[8]

"Bahá'u'lláh enjoined upon His followers to devote these days to feasting, rejoicing and charity. In a letter written on Shoghi Effendi's behalf it is explained that "the intercalary days [the five days before the fast] are specially set aside for hospitality, the giving of gifts, etc."[9]

WHO MUST FAST?

THERE ARE SOME EXEMPTIONS FROM FASTING, INCLUDING PEOPLE who are sick, traveling, children, the elderly, and people engaged in heavy labor.

"We have commanded you to pray and fast from the beginning of maturity; this is ordained by God, your Lord and the Lord of your forefathers. He hath exempted from this those who are weak from illness or age, as a bounty from His Presence, and He is the Forgiving, the Generous."[10]

According to Bahá'u'lláh, fasting begins when a child is mature enough to be spiritually responsible. This age is fifteen years old. The age when the elderly are exempt is seventy years old, regardless of their state of health.[11]

"Fasting is enjoined on all the believers once they attain the age of 15 and until they reach the age of 70 years." [12]

Women who are menstruating are also exempt. Bahá'u'lláh encourages her to pray and perform ablutions during this time instead.

"God hath exempted women who are in their courses from obligatory prayer and fasting. Let them, instead after performance of their ablutions, give praise unto God[.]"[13]

Finally, people who are traveling, sick people, women who are pregnant or breastfeeding are also exempt. "The traveller, the ailing, those who are with child or giving suck, are not bound by the Fast; they have been exempted by God as a token of His grace. He, verily, is the Almighty, the Most Generous.

"These are the ordinances of God that have been set down in the Books and Tablets by His Most Exalted Pen. Hold ye fast unto His statutes and commandments, and be not of those who, following their idle fancies and vain imaginings, have clung to the standards fixed by their own selves, and cast behind their backs the standards laid down by God. Abstain from food and drink from sunrise to sundown, and beware lest desire deprive you of this grace that is appointed in the Book."[14]

People engaged in heavy labor are also exempt but their meals should be simple and private out of respect for God.

"This exemption is also extended to people who are engaged in heavy labour, who, at the same time, are advised 'to show respect to the law of God and for the exalted station of the Fast' by eating 'with frugality and in private' [. . .]. Shoghi Effendi has indicated that the types of work which would exempt people from the Fast will be defined by the Universal House of Justice."[15]

Bahá'u'lláh revealed the length of a journey that may exempt the traveler from fasting and when and how to resume fasting when the journey is over.

"Should the traveller stop in a place, anticipating that he will stay there for no less than one month by the Bayán reckoning, it is incumbent on him to keep the Fast; but if for less than one month, he is exempt from fasting. If he arriveth during the Fast at a place where he is to stay one month according to the Bayán, he should not observe the Fast till three days have elapsed, thereafter keeping it throughout the remainder of its course; but if he come to his home, where he hath heretofore been permanently resident, he must commence his fast upon the first day after his arrival."[16]

People who are traveling are free to fast if they choose:

"Shoghi Effendi has clarified that while travellers are exempt from fasting, they are free to fast if they so wish. He also indicated that the exemption applies during the whole period of one's travel, not just the hours one is in a train or car, etc."[17]

Thus, fasting is an ancient practice that is also historically religious in nature. The end result is physical and spiritual health. In the next chapter we shall explore the true frontier of dietary medicine, Bahá'u'lláh's *Tablet to a Physician*.

---

1. Bahá'u'lláh, *The Kitáb-i-Aqdas: The Most Holy Book*, (Haifa: Bahá'í World Centre, 1992), 24-25.
2. Ibid, 179, n. 32.
3. Ibid.
4. *Bahá'í Prayers For Women: Selections from the Writings of Bahá'u'lláh, the Báb, 'Abdu'l-Bahá and the Greatest Holy Leaf*, (Los Angeles: Kalimát Press, 2000), 72.
5. Bahá'u'lláh, *The Kitáb-i-Aqdas*, 176-77, n. 25.
6. Ibid 177, n. 26.
7. Ibid, 25.
8. Ibid.
9. Ibid 178-179, n. 29.
10. Ibid, 22-23.
11. Ibid, 171, n. 14.
12. Ibid, 177, n. 25.
13. Ibid, 23.
14. Ibid, 25.
15. Ibid, 179, n. 31.
16. Ibid, 114, question 22.
17. Ibid, 179, n. 30.

6

GOD: THE DIVINE PHYSICIAN

The Tablet to a Physician is a tablet Bahá'u'lláh addressed to a doctor. Bahá'u'lláh addressed this tablet to a doctor who was well versed in ancient eastern medicine. The tablet is steeped in language from this ancient system that its recipient would have understood.[1] In this tablet, Bahá'u'lláh explains that diet is one way to cure disease. Bahá'u'lláh also appears to mention herbalism as a form of medical care.

"O God! The Supreme Knower! The Ancient Tongue speaks that which will satisfy the wise in the absence of doctors. O People, do not eat except when you are hungry. Do not drink after you have retired to sleep. Exercise is good when the stomach is empty; it strengthens the muscles. When the stomach is full it is very harmful. Do not neglect medical treatment, when it is necessary, but leave it off when the body is in good condition. Do not take nourishment except when (the process of) digestion is completed. Do not swallow until you have thoroughly masticated your food. Treat disease first of all through diet, and refrain from medicine. If you can find what you need for healing in a single herb do not use a compound medicine. Leave off medicine when the health is good, and use it in case of necessity.

When you begin to eat, begin with My Name El Abhá, and finish with the Name of God the Possessor of the Throne and the earth."[2]

Bahá'u'lláh then goes into more detail on what to do with food that is served. He says that "diametrically opposed foods" should not be mixed:

"If two diametrically opposite foods are put on the table do not mix them. Be content with one of them. Take first the liquid food before partaking of solid food. The taking of food before that which you have already eaten is digested is dangerous....

"When you have eaten walk a little that the food may settle. That which is difficult to masticate is forbidden by the wise. Thus the Supreme Pen commands you. A light meal in the morning is as a light to the body. Avoid all harmful habits: they cause unhappiness in the world.

"Search for the causes of disease. This saying is the conclusion of this utterance."[3]

In the Kitáb-i-Badi, Bahá'u'lláh gives more guidance on how much to eat and the quality of the food.

"In all circumstances they should conduct themselves with moderation; if the meal be only one course this is more pleasing in the sight of God; however, according to their means, they should seek to have this single dish be of good quality."[4]

There is more. It appears that this ancient system of medicine that Bahá'u'lláh speaks of was essentially a global system with few variances by region, as explained by Matthew Wood in his book, *The Book of Herbal Wisdom*.[5] In the West, this system spoke of the "humors" or "elements" of the body. This realm of ancient medicine is called "energetics."[6] The humors are essentially "patterns in psychological and physiological qualities" in the human body that must be in proportion to one other.[7] A person may achieve this proportionality through plant foods and herbal medicine. Each plant has its own energy signature or imprint that transfers to the person who consumes it, thus affecting the balance of his or her humors. Thus, when Bahá'u'lláh says avoid eating two "diametrically opposed foods" in one meal, He may have been referring to *yin* and *yang* foods under the corresponding energetic system. *Yin* and *yang* in the Chinese system, for example would mean the dual qualities "hot/cold," "light/dark," etc. As we shall see below, Bahá'u'lláh uses the word "humors" *and gives the correct proportion for each.*

Additionally, the humors are highly susceptible to human emotions. Thus, when Bahá'u'lláh reveals that "jealously eats the body" and "anger burns the liver," He may have been linking the emotions to the corresponding humors in the organs.[8] The "choleric liver" is called "wind" in the Chinese energetic system and its treatment protocols include numerous herbs.[9]

"Be content in all conditions, by this the person is preserved from a bad condition and from lassitude. Shun grief and sorrow, they cause the greatest misery. Say: Jealousy eats the body and anger burns the liver. Refrain from these two as you would avoid a lion."[10]

Further, Bahá'u'lláh references cleansing, which may be referring to the detox procedures that are becoming more and more popular today:

"To cleanse the body is essential, but only in temperate seasons (should it be done frequently). He who over-eats, his illness becomes more severe. We have arranged for each thing a cause and We have Bestowed upon it an effect. All this is from the Effulgence of My Name, which Influences everything. Your God is the Commander of all things. Say: From what We have explained, **the humors of the body** should not be excessive and their quantity depends upon the condition of the body. One sixth of each sixth part in its normal condition (is the right proportion)."[11]

Thus, Bahá'u'lláh appears to be referencing a system of energetics that contains six humors, which is one more than the Chinese system. He prescribes the exact proportion of each, "One sixth of each sixth part."[12]

Could this be the revival of an ancient system that will again predominate? Could this be the end of medicine as we know it and the beginning of natural health through diet and advanced herbalism? Only the future will tell.

THE BAHÁ'Í FAITH PROPHECIES THE BEGINNING OF A NEW ERA IN human history. After this time of turmoil, there will be peace, tranquility, and the end of war. Globally, there will be abundant food for all, medical care for all, education for all, a universal language, and universal justice system. Humanity will be healed by the grace of God.

We now have the template for the human diet in the Bahá'í Writings and the key to a healing system.

---

1. *Majmu'a-yi Alwah-i Mubaraka,* (Wilmette: Bahá'í Publishing Trust, 1981).
2. Bahá'u'lláh, Star of the West, vol. 13, no. 9, December 1922, p. 252.
3. Ibid.
4. Compiled by the Research Department of The Universal House of Justice, *Health and Healing*, (New Delhi: Bahá'í Publishing Trust, 2004), 2.
5. Wood, *The Book of Herbal Wisdom*, 33.
6. Matthew Wood, *The Practice of Traditional Western Herbalism: Basic Doctrine, Energetics, and Classification*, (Berkeley: North Atlantic Books, 2004), 9.
7. Ibid.
8. Bahá'u'lláh, *Tablet of Medicine*, originally revealed as "Lawh-i-Tibb" first written or published 1870.
9. Wood, *The Book of Herbal Wisdom*, 92.
10. Bahá'u'lláh, *Tablet of Medicine*.
11. Ibid.
12. Ibid.

www.ingramcontent.com/pod-product-compliance
Lightning Source LLC
Chambersburg PA
CBHW071141280326
41935CB00010B/1317